ACUPRESSURE MADE SIMPLE FOR YOURSELF:

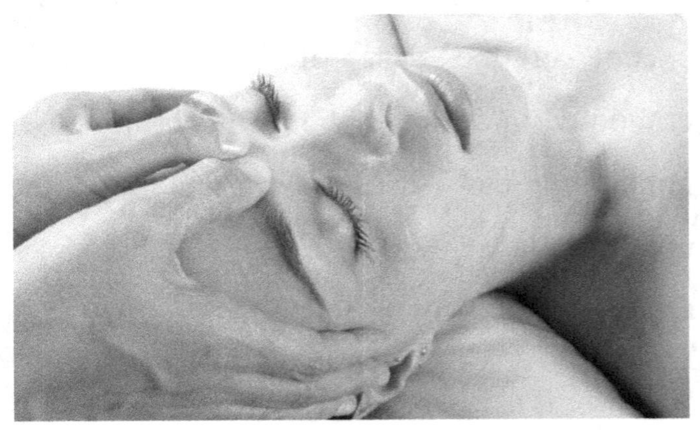

The Ultimate Guide To Easy Self-Treatment For Common Ailments

Robert S. Pinkson

Table of Contents

INTRODUCTION

Once upon a time, there was a wise old man who lived in a small village in China. He had spent his entire life studying the human body and its natural healing powers. The old man believed that the human body could heal itself if given the right tools and guidance.

One day, a young woman from the village came to the old man with a problem. She had been experiencing chronic headaches for years, and no matter what she did, the pain wouldn't go away. The woman had tried countless remedies and treatments, but nothing seemed to work.

The old man listened carefully to the woman's story, and then he gently placed his hands on her forehead and began to apply pressure to certain points on her face and head. The woman felt a strange sensation, almost like a release, as the old man continued to apply pressure.

After a few minutes, the old man removed his hands and told the woman to rest for a while. To her surprise, the woman realized that her headache was gone! She felt an immense sense of relief and gratitude towards the old man, and she wanted to learn more about this mysterious healing technique.

The old man explained that what he had used was a form of therapy called acupressure. Acupressure is an ancient healing technique that has been used in traditional Chinese medicine for thousands of years. It involves applying pressure to specific points on the body to stimulate the body's natural healing process.

The concept behind acupressure is that the human body has a network of meridians or energy channels that run throughout the body. These channels connect different parts of the body and are responsible for the flow of energy or "chi." When the flow of energy is disrupted, it can result in pain, illness, or other health problems.

Acupressure works by applying pressure to specific points along these meridians to restore the flow of energy and promote healing. The pressure can be applied using fingers, hands, elbows, or even special tools like acupressure mats.

Acupressure is a safe and non-invasive form of therapy that can be used to treat a wide range of health issues, including headaches, back pain, insomnia, and anxiety. It can also be used as a form of preventative medicine to maintain overall health and well-being.

Whether you're dealing with a specific health issue or simply looking to improve your overall well-being, acupressure can be a powerful tool to add to your toolkit.

CHAPTER 1

What is Acupressure?

Acupressure is an alternative healing technique that involves applying pressure to specific points on the body to stimulate energy flow and promote healing. It is based on the principles of Traditional Chinese Medicine (TCM) and is similar to acupuncture, except that it uses finger pressure instead of needles.

The philosophy behind acupressure is that the body has a network of energy channels, or meridians, which are linked to different organs and systems in the body. When these channels become blocked, it can result in physical and emotional imbalances. Acupressure aims to unblock these channels and restore balance to the body.

Traditional Chinese Medicine and Acupressure
Acupressure is based on Traditional Chinese Medicine (TCM), which is a holistic healing system that has been practiced in China for over 2,000 years. According to TCM theory, the body is composed of energy channels, or meridians, through which life force energy (known as Qi) flows. When the flow of Qi is disrupted, it can lead to disease or pain. Acupressure is a way to stimulate the flow of Qi and promote healing.

Understanding Pressure Points

Pressure points are specific points on the body that, when stimulated with pressure, can produce therapeutic effects. These points are located along the body's energy meridians, which are pathways of energy that flow throughout the body.

Understanding pressure points is an essential part of several healing therapies, including acupressure, acupuncture, and reflexology. These therapies use pressure points to help alleviate pain, improve circulation, and promote overall well-being.

Here are some essential facts to understand about pressure points:

LOCATION: Pressure points are located all over the body, from the head down to the feet. Each point corresponds to a specific organ or body part and has its unique function.

FUNCTION: Pressure points work by stimulating the body's natural healing response. Applying pressure to specific points can help to release tension, improve circulation, and reduce pain and inflammation.

ACUPRESSURE AND ACUPUNCTURE: Acupressure and

acupuncture are two therapies that use pressure points to promote healing. Acupressure involves using finger pressure to stimulate points, while acupuncture involves inserting fine needles into specific points.

REFLEXOLOGY: Reflexology is another therapy that uses pressure points. It involves applying pressure to specific points on the feet, hands, and ears, which are believed to correspond to different organs and systems in the body.

SAFETY: It is essential to use caution when applying pressure to pressure points. While acupressure and reflexology are generally safe, some points should be avoided during pregnancy or if you have certain health conditions. Always consult with a qualified practitioner before trying any therapy.

SELF-CARE: There are several pressure points that you can stimulate at home to promote relaxation and relieve stress. These include the "Third Eye" point between the eyebrows, the "Union Valley" point on the hand, and the "Bubbling Spring" point on the foot

How to make Acupressure Works for you?

Acupressure is a traditional healing technique that involves applying pressure to specific points on the body to alleviate pain, improve circulation, and promote overall well-being. Here are some tips on how to make acupressure work for you:

CONSULT WITH A PROFESSIONAL: Before starting any acupressure treatment, it is important to consult with a professional acupressurist. They will be able to assess your health condition and recommend the right acupressure points to target.

KNOW THE ACUPRESSURE POINTS: Familiarize yourself with the acupressure points that are relevant to your health condition. There are hundreds of acupressure points throughout the body, each with its unique function. Learn the location and function of the points that you need to target.

APPLY PRESSURE CORRECTLY: When applying pressure to an acupressure point, use your fingertips, knuckles, or elbows, depending on the location of the point. Apply firm, steady pressure for at least 30 seconds. Gradually increase the pressure until you feel a deep ache or tingling sensation.

BREATHE DEEPLY: Deep breathing can help you relax and focus while applying pressure to acupressure points. Take slow, deep breaths while applying pressure, and exhale slowly. This will help to release tension and promote relaxation.

BE PATIENT: Acupressure is not a quick fix. It may take several sessions before you start to see significant improvements in your health condition. Be patient and consistent with your treatments.

PRACTICE SELF-CARE: Acupressure is just one aspect of self-care. Eating a healthy diet, getting regular exercise, and getting enough sleep are all important for maintaining overall health and well-being.

KEEP AN OPEN MIND: Acupressure is a complementary therapy that works in conjunction with conventional medicine. Keep an open mind and be willing to try

different techniques and approaches to find
what works best for you

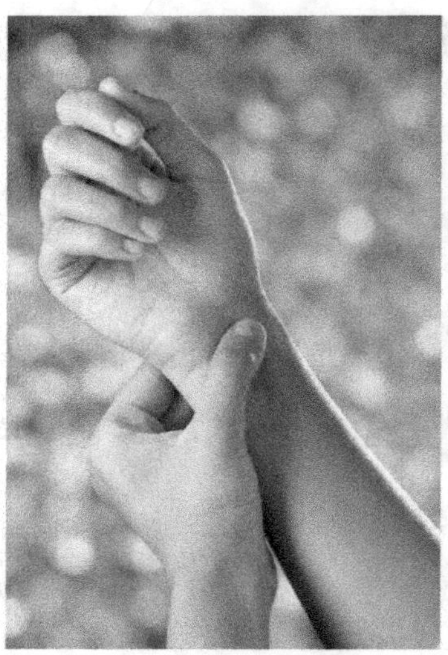

CHAPTER 2

Preparing for an Acupressure Session

Preparing for an acupressure session can help ensure that you get the most out of your treatment. Whether you are working with a professional acupressure practitioner or practicing self-acupressure at home, here are some tips to help you prepare for your session:

SET A GOAL

Before your acupressure session, take a few moments to set a goal for what you hope to achieve. This could be anything from reducing stress and anxiety to relieving physical pain or promoting overall wellness. By setting a goal, you create a sense of focus and purpose for your session.

CHOOSE A QUIET AND RELAXING ENVIRONMENT.

Acupressure is most effective when you are in a quiet and relaxing environment. If you are working with a professional acupressure practitioner, they will likely provide a calm and peaceful setting for your session. If you are practicing self-acupressure at home, create a quiet and relaxing space where you can focus on your treatment without distractions.

WEAR COMFORTABLE CLOTHING.

Wearing loose, comfortable clothing can help you relax and feel more comfortable during your acupressure session. Avoid wearing tight or restrictive clothing that could interfere with the flow of Qi through your body's meridians.

AVOID EATING A HEAVY MEAL BEFOREHAND

Eating a heavy meal before an acupressure session can interfere with digestion and make it more difficult for your body to absorb the benefits of the treatment. Instead, eat a light meal or snack a few hours before your session.

COMMUNICATE OPENLY WITH YOUR PRACTITIONER.

If you are working with a professional acupressure practitioner, be sure to communicate openly about any health concerns or symptoms you are experiencing. This will help your practitioner tailor your treatment to your specific needs and ensure that you get the most out of your session.

PRACTICE RELAXATION TECHNIQUES BEFORE YOUR SESSION.

To help prepare your body and mind for acupressure, practice relaxation techniques such as deep breathing, meditation, or gentle yoga. This can help you feel more relaxed and focused during your session, allowing you to fully benefit from the treatment.

STAY HYDRATED.

Drinking plenty of water before and after your acupressure session can help to support the body's natural healing processes and flush out toxins. Aim to drink at least 8-10 glasses of water throughout the day.

How To Locate Important Pressure Points

Locating pressure points is essential for anyone looking to use acupressure, acupuncture, or reflexology as a form of therapy. While some points can be easy to find, others may require some practice to locate them correctly. Here are some tips for locating important pressure points:

CONSULT A CHART: There are numerous charts available online and in books that can help you identify pressure points. These charts show the location of each point, along with a brief description of its function.

FEEL FOR TENDERNESS: Many pressure points are located in areas that may be tender to the touch. When applying pressure to an area, pay attention to any discomfort or tenderness you feel. These sensations can be a sign that you have found the correct point.

USE YOUR FINGERS: The easiest way to locate pressure points is to use your fingers. Start by applying gentle pressure to an area and gradually increase the pressure until you feel a slight ache or tenderness.

FOLLOW THE MERIDIANS: Pressure points are located along the body's energy meridians. These meridians are pathways of energy that flow throughout the body. Following the meridian lines can help you locate the pressure points along those pathways.

USE LANDMARKS: Some pressure points are located near specific landmarks on the body, such as bones or muscles. Using these landmarks as a guide can help you locate the correct point.

SEEK GUIDANCE: If you are having trouble locating a specific pressure point, consider seeking guidance from a qualified practitioner. A trained acupuncturist or reflexologist can help you find the correct points and provide guidance on how to stimulate them safely.

CHAPTER 3: ACUPRESSURE FOR COMMON AILMENTS

Headache and Migraine

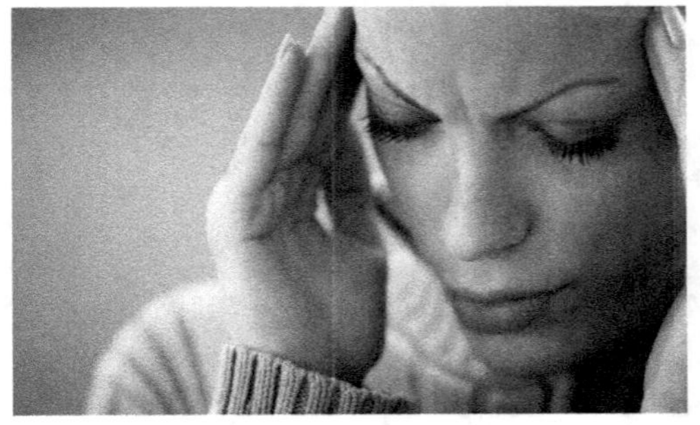

YIN TANG (THIRD EYE POINT)

LOCATION: Situated at the point where the bridge of the nose meets the forehead, within the depression between the eyebrows.

DIRECTION: To stimulate this point, use your index fingers to apply gentle pressure and massage in a circular motion for 1-2 minutes. You can also use your fingertips to tap on this point gently for 1-2 minutes. Some people find it helpful to take deep breaths while stimulating this point to help calm the mind and relax the body.

GB14 (GALLBLADDER 14)

LOCATION: This point is located on the forehead, in the depression directly above the center of each eyebrow. To locate it, place your fingers on the center of each eyebrow and slide them upward towards the hairline until you feel a small notch in the skull. GB14 is located in this notch.

DIRECTION:To stimulate this point, apply firm pressure with your index and middle fingers and massage in a circular motion for 2-3 minutes. You can also tap on this point gently with your fingertips for 1-2 minutes.

LI4 (LARGE INTESTINE 4)

LOCATION: This point is located on the back of the hand, in the webbing between the thumb and index finger. To locate it, place your thumb on the base of your index finger and slide it toward the webbing. LI4 is located at the highest point of the muscle when you bring your thumb and index finger close together.

DIRECTION: To stimulate this point, apply firm pressure with your thumb and massage in a circular motion for 2-3 minutes. You can also use your thumb to tap on this point gently for 1-2 minutes.

ST36 (STOMACH 36)

LOCATION: This point is located on the leg, about a hand's width below the bottom of the kneecap, on the outside of the leg. To locate it, place your hand just below your kneecap and locate the bony prominence on the outside of your leg. ST36 has located about one hand's width below this prominence, in a small depression between the shinbone and the muscle.

DIRECTION: To stimulate this point, apply firm pressure with your index and middle fingers and massage in a circular motion for

2-3 minutes. You can also use your thumb to press and hold this point for 1-2 minutes.

Neck pain and Tension

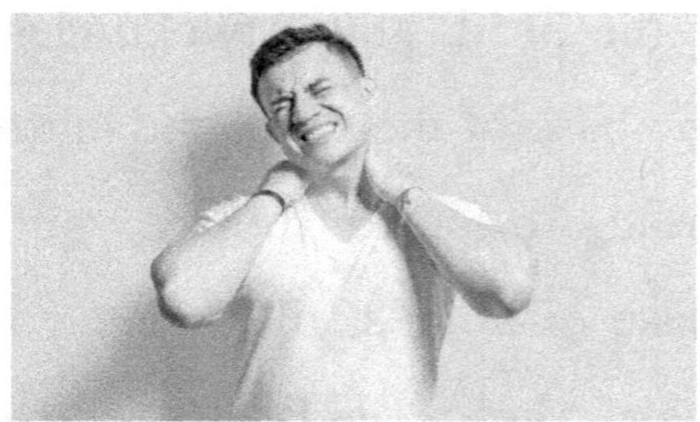

Neck pain is a common ailment that affects many people, especially those who spend long hours sitting at a desk or performing repetitive motions. Acupressure is a form of alternative medicine that involves applying pressure to specific points on the body to alleviate pain and promote healing. Here are the acupressure points for neck pain and tension

GV16 (GOVERNING VESSEL)

LOCATION: This point is located on the back of the head, about two finger widths above the base of the skull, and in the center of the head. To locate it, place your fingers at the base of your skull, where your neck meets your head, and then move them upward towards the top of your head until you feel a slight depression. This is the location of the GV16 point.

DIRECTION: To stimulate this point, use your fingertips to apply gentle pressure and massage in a circular motion for 1-2 minutes. You can also use your fingertips to tap on this point gently for 1-2 minutes. This point is often used to help relieve headaches and neck pain, as well as to promote relaxation and calmness.

LI4 (LARGE INTESTINE 4)

LOCATION: This point is located on the back of the hand, in the webbing between the thumb and index finger. To locate it, place your thumb on the base of your index finger and slide it toward the webbing. LI4 is located at the highest point of the muscle when you bring your thumb and index finger close together.

DIRECTION: To stimulate this point, use your thumb to apply firm pressure and massage in a circular motion for 1-2 minutes. You can also use your thumb to tap on this point gently for 1-2 minutes. However, it should be avoided during pregnancy as it may stimulate contractions.

Shoulder Pain and Tension

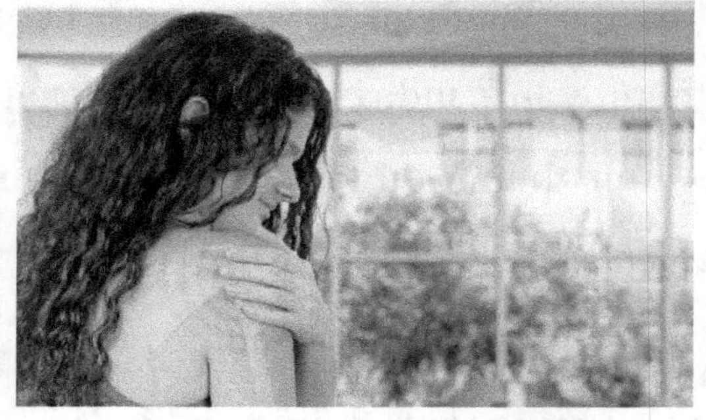

TW15

LOCATION: This point is located on the shoulder, midway between the base of the neck and the outer edge of the shoulder blade. To locate it, raise your arm to the side and locate the muscle bulge at the top of the shoulder. TW15 is located in the depression just below this bulge.

DIRECTION: To stimulate this point, use your fingertips or a massage ball to apply firm pressure and massage in a circular motion for 1-2 minutes. You can also use your fingertips to tap on this point gently for 1-2 minutes.

LI15 (LARGE INTESTINE 15)

LOCATION: This point is located on the shoulder, about three finger-widths below the top of the shoulder and on the outside of the upper arm. To locate it, find the bulge of the shoulder muscle and move your fingers down towards the elbow until you reach a depression. LI15 is located in this depression.

DIRECTION: To stimulate this point, use your fingertips or a massage ball to apply firm pressure and massage in a circular motion for 1-2 minutes. You can also use your fingertips to tap on this point gently for 1-2 minutes.

LI11 (LARGE INTESTINE 11)

LOCATION: This point is located on the outer side of the elbow crease. To locate it, bend your arm and locate the end of the crease on the outer side of your elbow. LI11 is located at the end of this crease.

DIRECTION: To stimulate this point, use your fingertips to apply firm pressure and massage in a circular motion for 1-2 minutes. You can also use your fingertips to tap on this point gently for 1-2 minutes.

GB21 (GALLBLADDER 21)

LOCATION: This point is located on the top of the shoulder, midway between the base of the neck and the outer edge of the shoulder blade. To locate it, find the muscle bulge at the top of the shoulder and move your fingers towards the neck until you feel a depression. GB21 is located in this depression.

DIRECTION: To stimulate this point, use your fingertips or a massage ball to apply firm pressure and massage in a circular motion for 1-2 minutes. You can also use your fingertips to tap on this point gently for 1-2 minutes. However, it should be avoided during pregnancy as it may stimulate contractions

Toothache

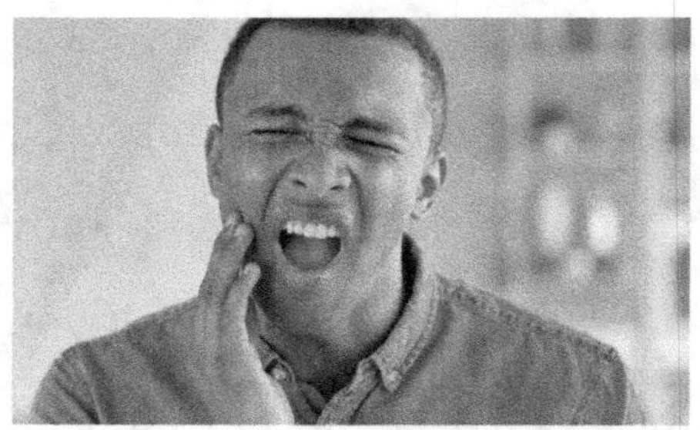

Toothache is a common condition that can be caused by a variety of factors, including tooth decay, gum disease, infection, or

injury. Here are the acupressure points for toothache

ST6 (STOMACH 6)

LOCATION: This point is located on the lower jaw, just in front of the earlobe and slightly below the cheekbone. To locate it, place your fingers on your jaw just in front of your earlobe and move them toward your mouth until you feel a slight depression. St6 is located in this depression.

ST3 (STOMACH 3)

LOCATION: This point is located on the cheek, directly below the pupil of the eye, and in line with the bottom of the nose. To locate it, find the depression on your cheekbone directly below your pupil and move your fingers toward your nose until you feel a slight depression. St3 is located in this depression.

DIRECTION (ST6 & ST3): To stimulate this point, use your fingertips to apply firm pressure and massage in a circular motion for 1-2 minutes. You can also use your fingertips to tap on this point gently for 1-2 minutes. Nonetheless, it is not advisable to use it during pregnancy as it has the potential to induce contractions.

Ear Pain

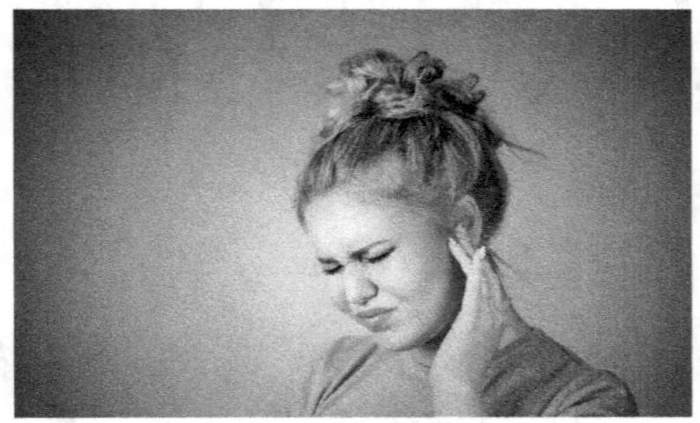

Ear pain can be a common problem that can occur due to various reasons, such as an infection, injury, or blockage in the ear canal. Here are some acupressure points for ear pain and how to perform acupressure to support ear health:

SI19 (SMALL INTESTINE 19)

LOCATION: This point is located in front of the ear, in the depression that is formed when you open your mouth. To locate it, open your mouth and locate the depression just in front of the ear canal. This depression houses the location of Si19.

GB2 (GALLBLADDER 2)

LOCATION: This point is located on the temple, in the depression between the outer corner of the eye and the eyebrow. To locate it, find the bony ridge of the eyebrow and move your fingers toward the outer corner of the eye. GB2 is located in the depression just below this ridge.

TW17 (TRIPLE WARMER 17)

LOCATION: This point is located behind the ear, in the depression at the base of the skull. To locate it, find the mastoid bone behind the ear and move your fingers upwards toward the base of the skull. TW17 is located in the depression just below this bone.

DIRECTION (SI19, GB2 & TW17): To stimulate this point, use your fingertips or a massage ball to apply firm pressure and massage in a circular motion for 1-2 minutes. You can also use your fingertips to tap on this point gently for 1-2 minutes.

Eye Pain

Acupressure is a natural and effective way to relieve eye pain and discomfort by stimulating specific acupressure points on the body that can promote blood flow and reduce tension in the eyes. Here are some points for eye pain and how to perform acupressure to support eye health.

TAI YANG

LOCATION: This point is located on the side of the head, in the depression that is formed between the ear and the eyebrow. To locate it, find the midpoint of the eyebrow and move your fingers toward the temple until you feel a slight depression. This depression is the location of Tai Yang.

DIRECTION: To stimulate this point, use your fingertips to apply firm pressure and massage in a circular motion for 1-2 minutes. You can also use your fingertips to tap on this point gently for 1-2 minutes.

LIV3 (LIVER 3)

LOCATION: This point is located on the top of the foot, between the big toe and the second toe. To locate it, find the depression between the two tendons on the top of your foot. Liv3 is located in this depression.

DIRECTION: To stimulate this point, use your thumb to apply firm pressure and massage in a circular motion for 1-2 minutes. You can also use your thumb to press and hold this point for 1-2 minutes. It is not advisable to use it during pregnancy.

Back Pain

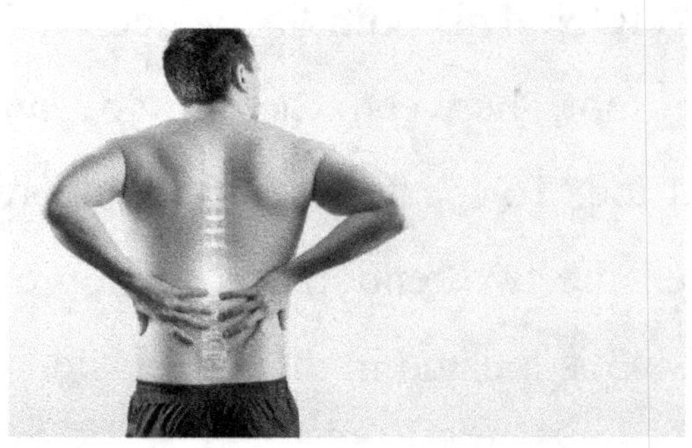

B27 (BLADDER 27)

LOCATION: This point is located in the lower back, at the level of the waist, and is approximately two finger widths from the spine on either side. To locate it, find the top of your hip bone (iliac crest) and move your fingers toward the middle of your back until you feel two bony protrusions. B27 is located just below these protrusions, on either side of the spine.

B34 (BLADDER 34)

LOCATION: This point is located in the buttock, on the back of the thigh, and is approximately four finger widths below the base of the buttock crease. To locate it, find the top of your buttock crease and move your fingers down toward the back of your thigh. B34 is located in the depression just below the bony prominence of the hip (greater trochanter).

B54 (BLADDER 54)

LOCATION: This point is located in the back of the knee, in the hollow that is formed when the knee is bent. To locate it, bend your knee and find the depression behind the knee joint. B54 is located in this depression, at the midpoint of the crease.

DIRECTION (B27, B34, B54): To stimulate this point, use your fingertips or a massage ball to apply firm pressure and massage in a circular motion for 1-2 minutes. You can also use your fingertips to tap on this point gently for 1-2 minutes.

Hip Pain

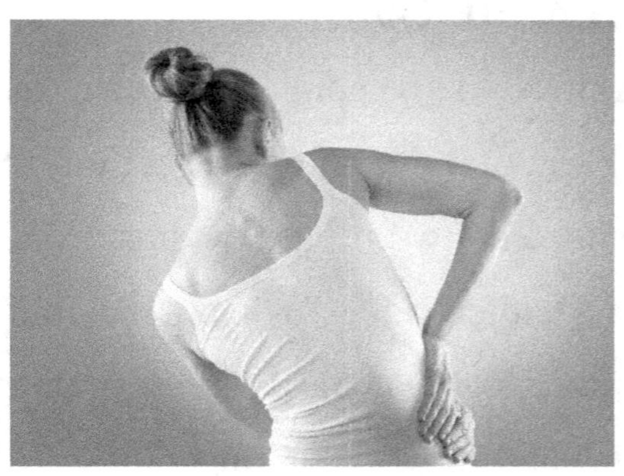

GB29 (GALLBLADDER 29)

LOCATION: This point is located on the outside of the hip, just below the hip joint. To locate it, find the bony prominence of the hip (greater trochanter) and move your fingers toward the front of your body until you feel a depression. GB29 is located in this depression.

B48 (BLADDER 48)

LOCATION: This point is located in the lower back, at the level of the sacrum, and is approximately two finger widths from the spine on either side. To locate it, find the bony protrusions at the base of your spine (sacrum) and move your fingers toward the sides of your body until you feel two bony protrusions. B48 is located just below these protrusions, on either side of the spine.

DIRECTION (GB29 & B48): To stimulate this point, use your fingertips or a massage ball to apply firm pressure and massage in a circular motion for 1-2 minutes. You can also use your fingertips to tap on this point gently for 1-2 minutes. This point is often used to help relieve lower back pain, sciatica, and pelvic pain, as well as to promote circulation and relieve tension in the lower back muscles.

Sore Throat

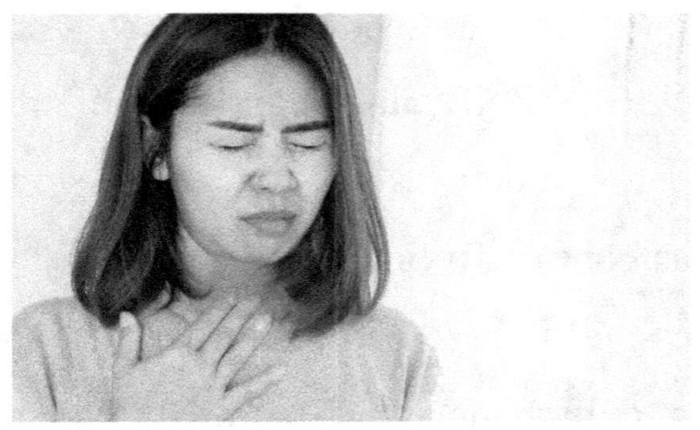

CV22 (CONCEPTION VESSEL)

LOCATION: This point is located at the bottom of the throat, in the center of the notch at the top of the breastbone. To locate it, place your fingers at the base of your throat, just above your collarbone, and slide them down until you feel the bony notch at the top of your breastbone. CV22 is located in the center of this notch.

K27 (KIDNEY 27)

LOCATION: These points are located on the front of the body, just below the collarbone and to either side of the sternum (breastbone). To locate them, place your fingers at the base of your throat, just above your collarbone, and slide them down towards your sternum until you feel two bony protrusions. K27 is located just below these protrusions, on either side of the sternum.

DIRECTION (CV22 & K27): To stimulate these points, use your fingertips to apply gentle pressure and massage in a circular motion for 1-2 minutes. You can also use your fingertips to tap on these points gently for 1-2 minutes. These points are often used to help relieve respiratory issues, such as coughing, chest congestion, and shortness of breath, as well as to promote relaxation and reduce stress and anxiety.

Sinusitis

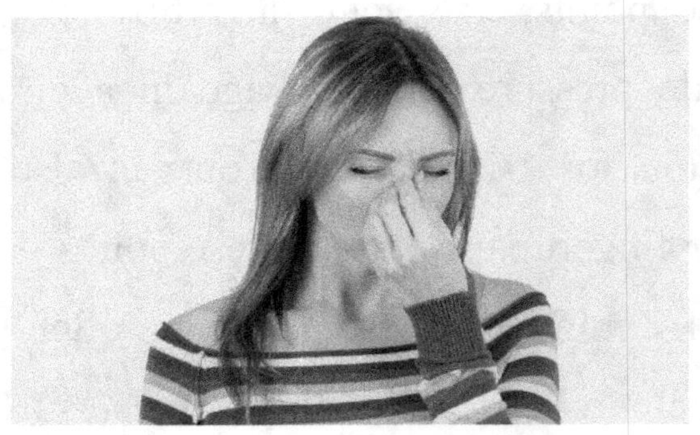

ST3 (STOMACH 3)

LOCATION: This point is located on the face, in the hollow just below the cheekbone, and to the side of the nose. To locate it, place your fingers on your cheekbone and slide them up towards your eye until you feel the hollow just below the bone. St3 is located in this hollow, about one finger width (about two centimeters) away from the side of the nose.

LI20 (LARGE INTESTINE 20)

LOCATION: This point is located on the face, at the bottom of the nose, and to either side of the nostrils. To locate it, place your fingers at the bottom of your nose, just above your upper lip, and slide them out towards your nostrils. Li20 can be found adjacent to each nostril.

B2 (BLADDER 2)

LOCATION: This point is located on the face, in the hollow just above the inner corner of each eye. To locate it, place your fingers at the inner corner of each eye and slide them up towards your eyebrows until you feel the hollow just above the inner corner. B2 is located in this hollow.

DIRECTION (ST3, LI20 & B2): To stimulate this point, use your fingertips to apply gentle pressure and massage in a circular motion for 1-2 minutes. You can also use your fingertips to tap on these points gently for 1-2 minutes.

Asthma

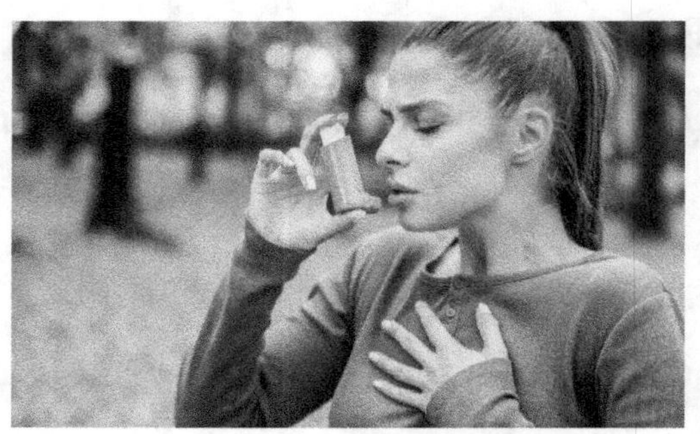

K27 (KIDNEY 27)

LOCATION: This point is located on the chest, in the groove between the collarbone and the first rib. To locate it, feel for the two bony protrusions at the base of your neck. K27 is located in the depression just below these protrusions, about one inch (2.5 cm) below the collarbone.

LU1 (LUNG 1)

LOCATION: This point is located on the chest, on the front of the body, in the depression below the collarbone, and beside the breastbone. To locate it, feel for the two bony protrusions at the base of your neck. Lu1 is located in the depression just below these protrusions, about one inch (2.5 cm) below the collarbone.

B13 (BLADDER 13)

LOCATION: This point is located on the back, in the space between the shoulder blades, at the level of the third thoracic vertebra. To locate it, stand or sit with your back straight and feel for the bony protrusions at the base of your neck. B13 is located at the same level as the third vertebra, about two inches (5 cm) away from the spine on either side.

DIRECTION (K27, LU1, & B13): To stimulate this point, use your fingertips or knuckles to apply firm pressure and massage in a circular motion for 1-2 minutes. You can also use a tennis ball or other round object to apply pressure to this point while lying on your back.

Insomnia and Sleep Problems

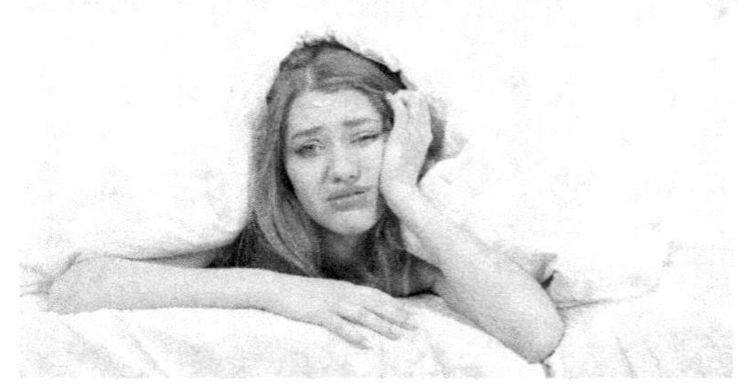

GB20 (GALL BLADDER 20)

LOCATION: This point is located on the back of the neck, in the hollows at the base of the skull. To locate it, find the two large muscle ridges at the back of your neck and feel for the hollows on either side of the spine, just below the base of the skull.

B10 (BLADDER 10)

LOCATION: This point is located on the back of the neck, about two finger widths below the base of the skull and on either side of the spine. To locate it, find the two large muscle ridges at the back of your neck and feel for the point where they meet the skull.

B38 (BLADDER 38)

LOCATION: This point is located on the lower back, about four finger widths below the waistline and two finger widths away from the spine on either side. To locate it, find the top of your hip bone and place your fingers on the muscles to either side of your spine, about four finger widths below the waistline.

DIRECTION (GB20, B10 & B38): To stimulate this point, use your fingertips to apply firm pressure and massage in a circular motion for 1-2 minutes. You can also use your fingertips to tap on this point gently for 1-2 minutes.

H7 (HEART 7)

LOCATION: This point is located on the inside of the wrist, on the crease where the wrist meets the hand. To locate it, place your hand palm up and find the crease on the inside of your wrist.

DIRECTION: To stimulate this point, use your thumb to apply firm pressure and massage in a circular motion for 1-2 minutes. You can also use your thumb to tap on this point gently for 1-2 minutes. This point is often used to help relieve anxiety, insomnia, and palpitations, as well as to promote relaxation and reduce stress

Hiccup

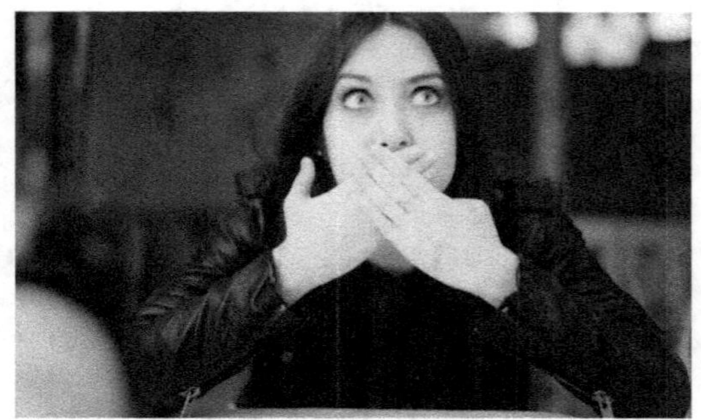

CV12 (CONCEPTION VESSEL)

LOCATION: This point is located on the front of the body, in the midline of the abdomen, about four finger widths (about eight centimeters) above the navel. To locate it, place your fingertips on the navel and slide them up towards the chest until you feel a slight depression in the midline of the abdomen. CV12 is located in this depression.

CV17 (CONCEPTION VESSEL 17)

LOCATION: This point is located on the front of the body, in the midline of the chest, at the level of the fourth intercostal space (between the fourth and fifth ribs). To locate it, place your fingertips on the center of the chest and slide them down towards the sternum (breastbone) until you feel a slight depression in the midline of the chest. CV17 is located in this depression.

DIRECTION (CV12 & CV17): To stimulate this point, use your fingertips to apply firm pressure and massage in a circular motion for 1-2 minutes. You can also use your fingertips to tap on this point gently for 1-2 minutes.

Angina and Palpitations

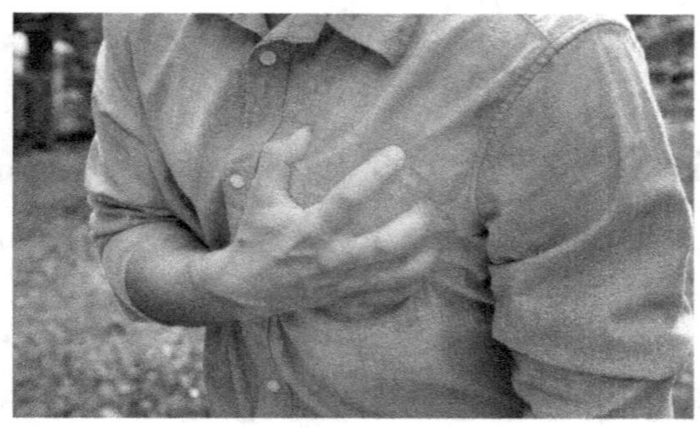

P6 (PERICARDIUM 6)

LOCATION: This point is located on the inside of the wrist, about two finger widths (about three centimeters) above the crease of the wrist, between the tendons of the forearm muscles. To locate it, place three fingers of one hand on the inside of the wrist of your other hand, just below the base of the palm. P6 is located in the middle of the three tendons that run parallel to each other.

H7 (HEART 7)

LOCATION: This point is located on the inside of the wrist, on the pinky side, about one finger width (about two centimeters) above the crease of the wrist. To locate it, place three fingers of one hand on the inside of the wrist of your other hand, just below the base of the palm. H7 is located on the radial side of the wrist, in the depression between the tendons of the forearm muscles.

DIRECTION (P6 & H7): To stimulate this point, use your fingertips to apply firm pressure and massage in a circular motion for 1-2 minutes. You can also use your fingertips to tap on this point gently for 1-2 minutes.

High Blood Pressure

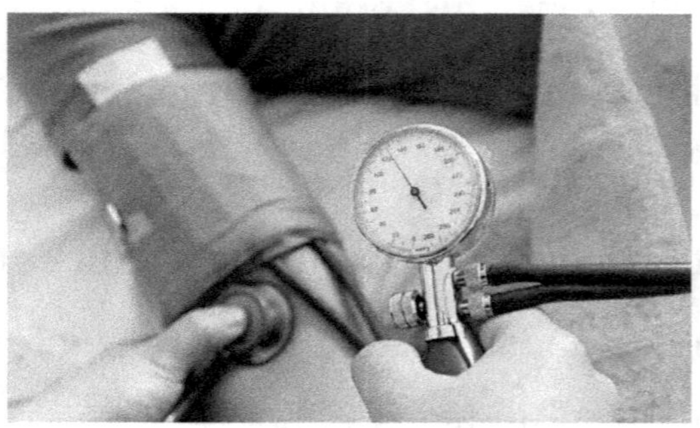

K3 (KIDNEY 3)

LOCATION: This point is located on the inside of the foot, in the depression between the ankle bone and the Achilles tendon. To locate it, feel for the highest point of the ankle bone and slide your finger down into the depression behind it. K3 is located at the point where your finger stops.

TW15

LOCATION: This point is located on the shoulder, midway between the base of the neck and the tip of the shoulder. To locate it, feel for the upper edge of the shoulder blade (scapula) and the collarbone (clavicle) and locate the point halfway between them.

DIRECTION (K3 & TW15): To stimulate this point, use your fingertips to apply firm pressure and massage in a circular motion for 1-2 minutes. You can also use your fingertips to tap on this point gently for 1-2 minutes. This point is often used to help relieve shoulder pain, stiffness, and tension, as well as to promote overall shoulder health and function.

Stomach Ache

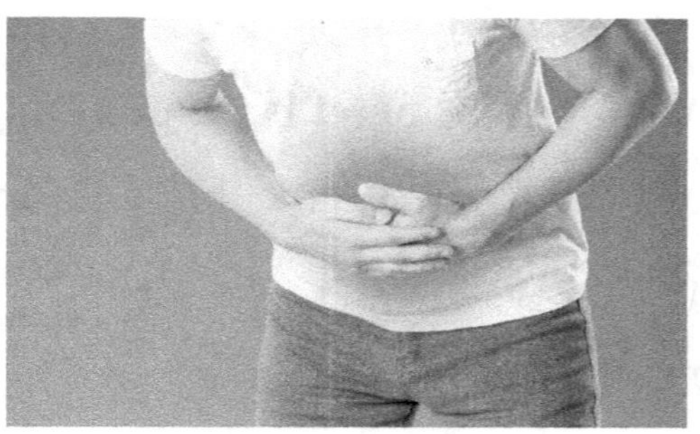

SP15 (SPLEEN 15)

LOCATION: This point is located on the inside of the thigh, about four finger widths (about eight centimeters) above the kneecap. To locate it, place your hand on your thigh so that your thumb is pointing towards your groin and your fingers are pointing towards your knee. SP15 is located on the inside of the thigh, at the point where your little finger rests.

LIV3 (LIVER 3)

LOCATION: This point is located on the top of the foot, between the big toe and the second toe. To locate it, place your hand on the top of your foot and slide your finger down between the bones of the big toe and second toe until you reach the point where they come together. Liv3 is located at the point where your finger rests.

CV6 (CONCEPTION VESSEL)

LOCATION: This point is located on the midline of the abdomen, two finger widths (about four centimeters) below the navel. To locate it, place your hand on your abdomen so that your little finger is resting on the pubic bone and your thumb is resting on the belly button. CV6 is located in the center of this space.

DIRECTION (SP15, LIV3 & CV6): To stimulate this point, use your fingertips to apply firm pressure and massage in a circular motion for 1-2 minutes. You can also use your fingertips to tap on this point gently for 1-2 minutes.

Nausea and Vomiting

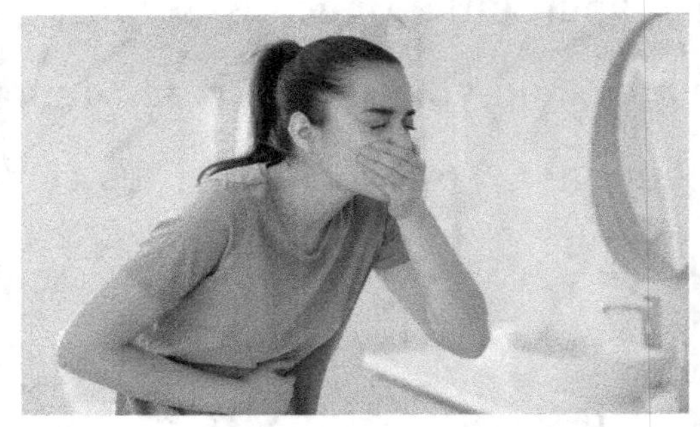

P6 (PERICARDIUM 6)

LOCATION: This point is located on the inside of the wrist, about two finger widths (about four centimeters) above the wrist crease. To locate it, place your hand palm up and use your thumb to locate the wrist crease. P6 is located two finger widths above the crease, between the tendons of the forearm muscles.

DIRECTION: To stimulate this point, use your fingertips or thumb to apply firm pressure and massage in a circular motion for 1-2 minutes. You can also use your fingertips or a wristband to apply continuous pressure to this point for several minutes.

Hot flashes

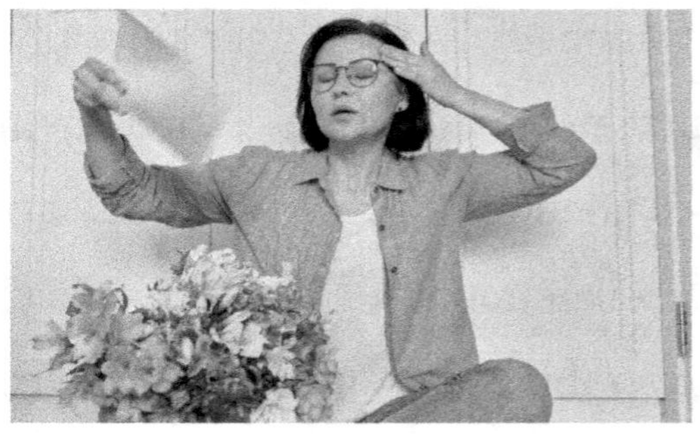

K1 (KIDNEY 1)

LOCATION: This point is located on the sole, at the depression where the ball of the foot meets the arch. To locate it, place your thumb on the inside edge of the ball of the foot and your index finger on the outside edge of the arch. K1 is located at the midpoint of this depression.

DIRECTION: To stimulate this point, use your thumb or index finger to apply firm pressure and massage in a circular motion for 1-2 minutes. You can also use a tennis ball or other round object to roll back and forth over this point for several minutes.

Urinary Retention

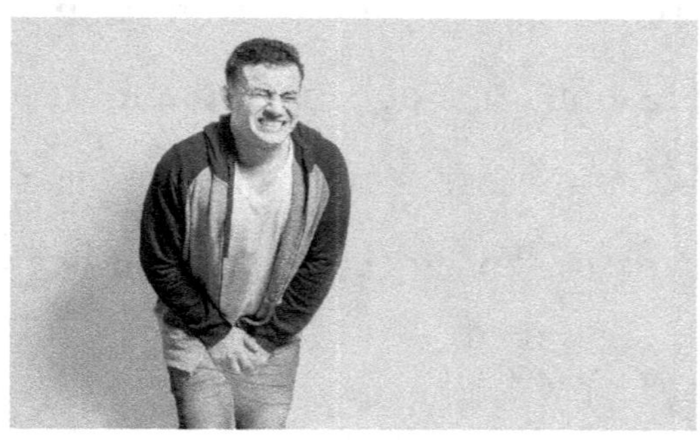

SP9 (SPLEEN 9)

LOCATION: This point is located on the inside of the lower leg, about three finger widths (about six centimeters) above the inner ankle bone. To locate it, place your hand on the inner ankle bone with your fingers pointing towards the knee. SP9 is located on the inside of the leg, at the point where your little finger rests.

DIRECTION: To stimulate this point, use your fingertips or knuckles to apply firm pressure and massage in a circular motion for 1-2 minutes. You can also use your fingertips to tap on this point gently for 1-2 minutes.

Skin Itching

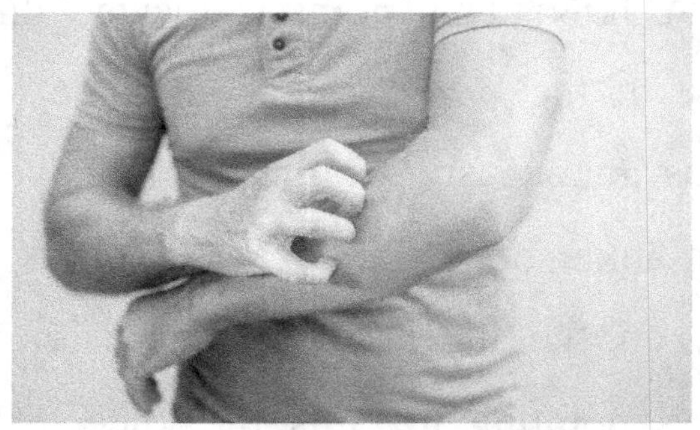

LI11 (LARGE INTESTINE 11)

LOCATION: This point is located on the outer end of the elbow crease, on the outer side of the arm. To locate it, bend your arm and look for the crease on the outer side of the elbow joint. Li11 is located at the end of this crease, closest to the wrist.

DIRECTION: To stimulate this point, use your fingertips or knuckles to apply firm pressure and massage in a circular motion for 1-2 minutes. You can also use a wristband or acupuncture needle to apply continuous pressure to this point for several minutes. This point is often used to help relieve pain and stiffness in the elbow and arm, reduce inflammation, and improve

immune function. It can also be helpful for
digestive issues and skin conditions.

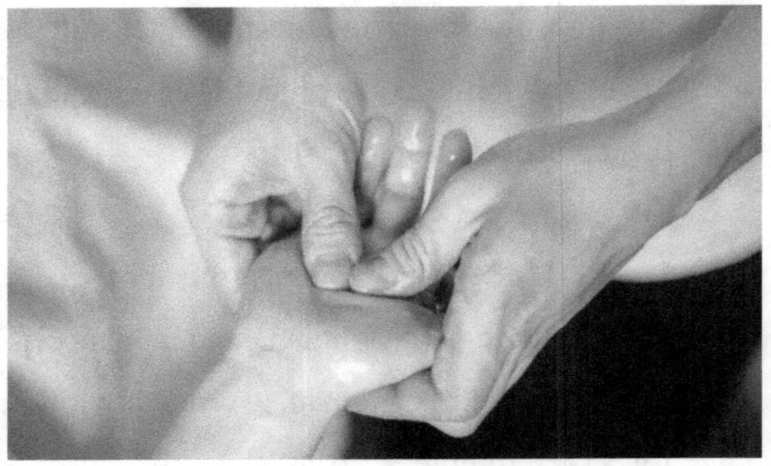

CHAPTER 4

Tips for Success with Acupressure

Acupressure is an ancient healing technique that involves the application of pressure to specific points on the body to promote relaxation, relieve pain, and improve overall health and well-being. Here are some tips for success with acupressure:

Learn about the pressure points: Acupressure involves applying pressure to specific points on the body, and it's important to know where these points are located and how to apply pressure correctly. You can learn about the pressure points from books, online resources, or from a qualified acupressure practitioner.

FIND A QUIET AND COMFORTABLE PLACE: To practice acupressure, you need a quiet and comfortable space where you won't be disturbed. This could be a quiet room in your home or a peaceful outdoor location.

PRACTICE DEEP BREATHING: Deep breathing can help you relax and prepare for acupressure. Take deep, slow breaths and focus on your breath as you prepare to apply pressure to the pressure points.

START WITH LIGHT PRESSURE: When you begin applying pressure to the pressure points, start with light pressure and gradually increase the pressure. Avoid applying too much pressure too quickly, as this can be painful and uncomfortable.

USE THE RIGHT AMOUNT OF PRESSURE: The amount of pressure you apply depends on your tolerance level and the sensitivity of the pressure point. Generally, a firm but gentle pressure is recommended.

FOCUS ON ONE PRESSURE POINT AT A TIME: To maximize the benefits of acupressure, it's best to focus on one pressure point at a time. Apply pressure to the point for 1-2 minutes, then move on to the next point.

BE PATIENT: Acupressure is not a quick fix, and it may take several sessions to see significant results. Be patient and consistent in your practice, and you will gradually start to see improvements in your health and well-being.

Acupressure For Specific Health Conditions Safety Consideration

Acupressure is a natural healing technique that has been used for thousands of years to treat a wide range of health conditions. However, it is important to use acupressure safely and responsibly, especially when treating specific health conditions. Here are some safety considerations to keep in mind when using acupressure:

CONSULT WITH A HEALTHCARE PROFESSIONAL: If you have a specific health condition or are unsure if acupressure is safe for you, it is important to consult with a healthcare professional before beginning acupressure therapy. They can help you determine the appropriate acupressure points and techniques for your specific needs and advise you on any potential risks or interactions with medications.

AVOID USING ACUPRESSURE ON OPEN WOUNDS OR AREAS WITH INFLAMMATION: If you have an open wound or an area of your body with inflammation or swelling, it is best to avoid using acupressure in that area, as it may exacerbate the condition and cause further discomfort.

USE GENTLE PRESSURE: Acupressure should be performed using gentle pressure, not forceful pressure. Applying too much pressure can cause pain, bruising, or even tissue damage.

AVOID USING ACUPRESSURE ON CERTAIN AREAS OF THE BODY: There are certain areas of the body where acupressure should be avoided, including the abdomen and lower back during pregnancy, as well as the neck and throat area, as there is a risk of damaging the carotid artery.

CONCLUSION

Acupressure Made Simple is a comprehensive guide that empowers you to take control of your health and well-being. By learning how to locate and stimulate key pressure points in your body, you can relieve pain, reduce stress, and promote relaxation safely and naturally.

The techniques presented in this book are simple and easy to understand, making acupressure accessible to everyone, regardless of their prior knowledge or experience. By incorporating acupressure into your daily routine, you can relieve stress, reduce pain, boost your immune system, and improve your overall quality of life. With practice and patience, you can become a master of acupressure and harness the power of this ancient healing art to transform your physical, emotional, and spiritual health.

So, whether you are a seasoned practitioner or just starting your journey with acupressure, this book is your go-to resource for all your self-care needs. With Acupressure Made Simple, you have the tools and knowledge to live a healthier, happier, and more fulfilling life.